THREE LIVES
OF

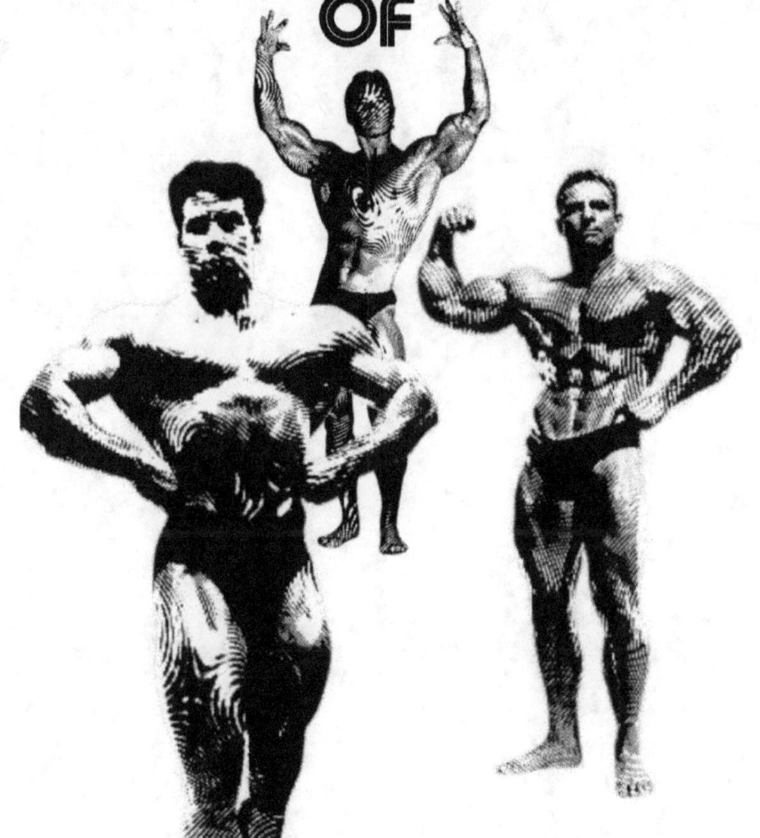

GOLDEN AGE
BODYBUILDERS

CONTENTS

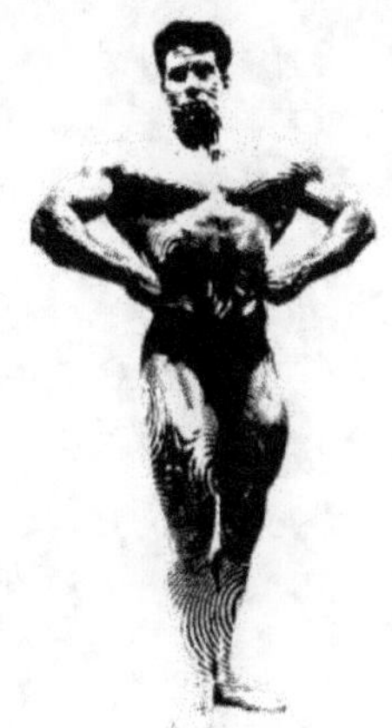

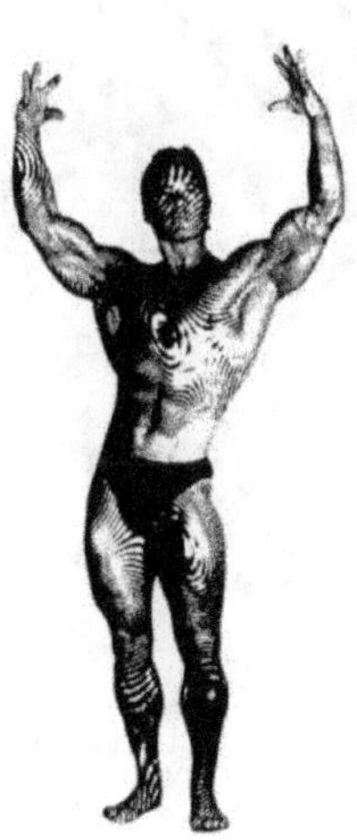

INTRODUCTION

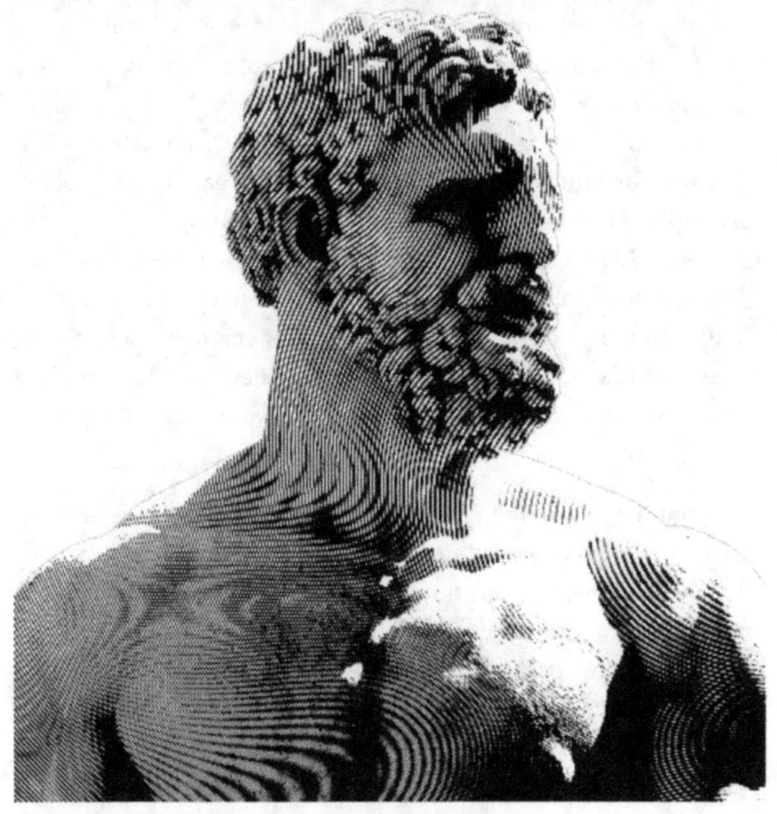

THE ENORMOUS CONDESCENSION OF POSTERITY

For the Romans, the purpose of writing and of studying history was quite clear. Whereas today we might expect an historian simply to tell things 'as they were', and leave the moral commentary out altogether, Roman history was by its very nature a moral enterprise; it was meant to edify and not just inform. It was a kind of 'monumental history', to use a term from Nietzsche's essay, 'On the Uses and Disadvantages of History for Life': stories that empower the reader with noble examples to emulate in the present. That's what the great historian Livy, beloved of Machiavelli, did. He told stories that showed how political virtue consisted of defending the Roman polity to the death, if need be, against its enemies. Even with later historians like Tacitus, who complicated the telling of the story by recounting far more of vice than of virtue, the moral purpose remained.

By contrast, we in the present have little faith in the ability of history to tell us anything other than 'the facts' of what happened once upon a time. Perhaps 'at best', for the Euro-American imperial and colonial powers, history is a catalogue of shame, to be used to justify endless hand-wringing, apologies and policies of affirmative action. Or the past is used selectively to confirm and justify our own preconceptions, political beliefs and ultimately our sense of superiority; witness, for instance, the urbanite Mary Beard wandering the streets of Rome, endlessly eulogising the benefits of the 'multicultural' ancient city. 'I just love the hustle and bustle of the big city, it's so DYNAMIC...' Despite the full-frontal assault that was waged on the notion of Progress in the twentieth century, old habits of thought die hard.

This condescending attitude is very clearly on display where the matter of health and fitness is concerned. Tweet that ancient diets and lifestyles might have been healthier or, heaven forbid, better than modern ones and wait for the flock of redditors to appear, darkening the sun. 'Yeah, you keep your massive infant mortality, rotting teeth, stunted growth and illiteracy thks. Ever heard of pre-eclampsia? LOL. Retard.' 'Yeah but did they have Netflix?' 'Raw milk? More like diarrhea and early death, sweety.' And so on, and so on, ad nauseam. Try reading Weston Price, *Nutrition and Physical Degeneration*, my midwit friends, and then James C. Scott, *Against the Grain*, for good measure: perhaps you'll learn something. The notion that ancient physical feats might have equalled or even bettered present attempts is usually greeted with the same mixture of incredulity and derision. But there is plenty of evidence to suggest that we really have been looking 'through the wrong end of the long telescope of Time', as D.H. Lawrence put it. A 1 058lb boulder discovered on the Greek island of Thera bears the inscription 'Eumastas, the son of Critobulus, lifted me from the ground.' Such a lift would not constitute a strict competition deadlift, for which Hafthor Bjornsson holds the world record of 1 104lb; but Hafthor was lifting a barbell and using straps, and the sheer difficulty of getting a hold of, let alone holding onto, a 1 058lb boulder would almost certainly make lifting it impossible for most if not all modern weightlifters. 'LOL. Eumastas probably just wrote that to make himself look good.' Maybe. But what would our midwit friends say about the following? In 2003, archaeologists discovered six sets of Ice Age footprints in a claypan lake bed in Australia which indicate that the men, who were probably running to outflank a prey animal, could easily have given the average elite Olympic sprinter a run for his money. One of these men, who probably stood 6′5″, was travelling at 23 mph – and this running barefoot through a muddy shallow lake. On a prepared running track, wearing modern shoes, this man would almost certainly have been able to better Usain Bolt's 27mph peak during the 100m dash. Perhaps these Chad antipodeans staged the whole scene, meticulously calculating the necessary stride distances to give the impression they were faster than the world's fastest man of twelve millennia hence. Or maybe, applying the principle of Occam's razor, they simply could run that fast, without the aid of Netflix or pasteurisation or hyperbaric chambers to aid their recovery. For many further examples, read *Manthropology*, by Peter McAllister.

If bodybuilding, the subject of this book, is simply about being able to boast the largest muscles possible, then of course today's bodybuilders are better than their predecessors: a straight line of 'progress' can be drawn from the sport's origins in the 1940s through to today. Q.E.D. But the 'mass monster' wasn't always the ideal, and since at least the 1980s competitors and observers have argued that bodybuilding lost its way when it sacrificed a proper sense of proportion and balance, the so-called 'Golden Ratio', for sheer physical size at any cost. Bodybuilders, while becoming larger and larger, have simultaneously receded from view as people. Larger than life only in physical proportions, bodybuilders spend their days in one of three places: the gym, the supermarket or at home, recovering from their workouts by huffing bland pre-prepared meals and protein shakes, and of course taking vast quantities of 'supplements'. A series of facile catchphrases that would shame a toddler with Tourette's or a handful of banal self-help maxims – this is now enough to constitute a 'character'. And as much as these men like to parade their physiques and pretend that they are Spartans or warriors, their bodies are good for little more than waddling behind a supermarket trolley, clearing the aisles of tuna, packets of rice and skimmed milk. When their professional careers end, these men are broken, physically and mentally. Look at Ronnie Coleman, barely able to walk, his greatest regret being two missed reps in an 800lb squat attempt; or Lee Priest, his face now covered in hideous tattoos.

The bodybuilders of the so-called Golden Age of bodybuilding (roughly from the late 1940s until the 1970s) aspired to a different kind of beauty and to a different kind of life, one that was not limited by the quantity of food one needed to consume or the hours of sleep that were required for MAXIMUM GAINZZZ. The three men who make up the subject of this book – Reg Park, Chuck Sipes and Chet Yorton – really were larger than life, men of great power who did much more than just build their bodies. Their lives offer ample instruction about how a beautiful body can be part of a beautiful life. The case of Chuck Sipes, in particular, at least for me, could not exemplify better the difference between our present one-dimensional muscle men and those of the past. After surviving a terrible parachuting accident while a member of the 82nd Airborne, Chuck set about building a massive, powerful physique, and within a short period of time was already winning bodybuilding competitions, as well as wowing audiences with displays of strength in the manner of the old-time strongmen. This he did at the same time as working as a lumberjack in the forests and sawmills of California, a lifestyle that would terrify the average bodybuilder or gymbro of today, so jealous of his rest time and anxious in the extreme not to compromise his gains with excess 'cardio'. But that was far from all there was to Chuck Sipes. He was also a talented banjo-picker, and a painter of detailed scenes from the Old West and American wilderness he loved so much. Most admirably of all, for decades he devoted much of his free time to mentoring troubled young men, the sort who had been abandoned not just by their families but by society itself. He helped them to turn their lives around and break the cycle of criminality. Chuck Sipes did not just look like a hero: he was one.

I chose biographies, and three of them, for a particular reason. Biography is an ancient form of moral exposition, as seen for instance in *Three Lives of Alcibiades, Dion and Atticus*, by Cornelius Nepos. By its very form, biography offers a powerful means for instruction. For biography reveals the true structure of a life in relation to death. Contrary to what post-modern philosophers and literary critics have to say about the death of meta-narrative and even the death of narrative altogether, the structure of narrative is built in to life: every life, without fail, has a beginning, a middle and an end. To put it another way, you could say that every life has the form of a quest, within which are nested multiple smaller quests, some of a narrower, more local meaning and others meaningful only within the whole. By narrating a man's life, the fruits of his actions are revealed and shown, in the final instance, for what they are, good and bad, and how they relate to one another. Every man's quest ends in the same place – death's other kingdom – but what happens in between is anyone's guess. For some, there is only vain, directionless striving – their lives appear like Brownian motion, the random movement of particles, before they are snuffed out – but for others, men of power, there is direction, coherence, purpose – triumph.

It should be noted that, while Reg Park and Chuck Sipes are both dead, Chet Yorton is still alive; although it is difficult to come by any reliable information about his current activities or whereabouts. Chet is by far the most enigmatic of the three men, whereas Reg has had a huge amount of ink devoted to his life and achievements since his appearance on the scene at the end of the 1940s; Chuck is somewhere in between. This disparity will of course be reflected in the detail and the structure of the biographies as they are told. While many of you may be familiar with Reg Park, my intention with Chuck and with Chet is as much to raise awareness of these unfairly neglected men as it is simply to chronicle their deeds.

As well as recalling these men's lives and achievements, I have included detailed, although not exhaustive, discussion of their routines and diets. Contrary to what somebody with a crude notion of progress within the sport might believe, these men were not somehow 'less well informed' about how to build muscle, simply because they had less than say Dorian Yates or Kai Greene. Rather, like Alex Jones, these men were pioneers and explorers, never afraid to experiment and ultimately to reflect upon and be critical of their training. To them we owe some of our fundamental approaches, such as the 5x5, and they also foreshadowed many of today's health and fitness crazes, such as ketogenic dieting and even fasting. These routines are not museum pieces or curiosities, to be wondered at, but cues for your own training and approach to the question of muscle-building. As I've said before, elsewhere, there is no single way.

So, for those wanting to build a body in service of life, rather than dedicate their life to the service of a body, I give you: Reg Park, Chuck Sipes and Chet Yorton. Let the monuments of their lives inspire you to great deeds.

A NOTE ON STEROID USE

Before I begin, it's worth discussing the issue of steroid use in a little depth. All three of the bodybuilders in this book spoke out prominently against steroids, at a time when their use among physique competitors and sportsmen was becoming more and more common. Chuck and Chet, in particular, staked their entire reputations on the claim that they had never and would never take steroids. Chuck retired completely from competition in the early seventies, after penning an article in *Muscle Training* magazine in which he claimed that 'drugs are destroying muscle men'. Chet retired from mainstream competition to form his own *Natural Bodybuilder's Association*, in 1975.

For many, the claim that any of these men was not on steroids will seem fantastical. Consider the learned opinions of r/nattyorjuice on Chet Yorton, for instance. 'Chet is full of schet.' 'Liar and gay.' And, most damningly of all, 'Looks like Mike O'Hearn's dad'. Not one voice is offered, at least not unironically, in support of his claim. u/samiam702 admits that Chet may have 'one in a million genetics', but since only an

African American could have such, ergo Chet must secretly be African American. So we wuz Chet Yorton too now, huh?

In the case of Reg Park, Nattyornot.com uses the following actual reasoning to arrive at the claim that Reg Park was unlikely to be a natty.

- Steroids were available ten years before Reg won his first show, in 1949. Testosterone was synthetically produced for the first time in 1935, and testosterone propinionate was first mentioned in a letter to the editor of *Strength and Health* in 1938.
- Reg was at times as large as if not larger than Arnold, an admitted steroid user.
- Reg competed in untested shows.
- Reg was the first bodybuilder to bench 500lb. Ed Coan, the famous powerlifter, pressed 584lb at a similar weight to Reg. Coan was an enhanced lifter.

For many, even in the absence of definitive evidence (drug tests or personal admissions), this line of argument will be enough to convict not just Reg but also Chuck and Chet of steroid use. All three men were massive and massively strong.

Consider the following, though. First, the fact that in the early days of bodybuilding there just wasn't the same stigma that would later be attached to steroid use. Neither Chuck nor Chet had quite the same incentive that today's 'natty' lifters have to speak out in the way they did: no reputation (beyond their own self-respect), no Instagram or Youtube subscribers, no sponsorship deals were at stake for them. Chuck actually abandoned competition as a result of his stance on steroids, and speaking out against steroids and immoral behaviour did Chet's career no good whatsoever. Secondly, Chuck and Chet's rage against steroids makes much less sense against the background of two physiques built by furtive steroid use than it does against the background of two physiques built out of tragedy through vision and sheer force of will. Both men survived terrible accidents, only to shed their broken bodies and become physique champions within a period of a few years. Wouldn't you be angry to see your competition – of whom Chet in particular had a very low moral estimation – reach the same heights as you, with only a fraction of the pain and suffering, and the aid of synthetic growth factors?

Ultimately, it's up to you to decide. For me, at least, everything about these three men and their stories says that they were special, physically – and morally. When you read these stories, I'm confident you'll think so too.

N.B. At the time I wrote *Three Lives of Golden Age Bodybuilders*, the great Chet Yorton was still alive. Sadly, 'late' is now an epithet that must be added to 'great'. On 7 November 2020, Chet discovered the lifeless body of his wife Vicky, at home. The shock was apparently enough to kill him; he died of a heart attack. Husband and wife were together in death, as they had been in life.

Tributes to this legend of Golden Age bodybuilding poured in, although the news took some time to spread. Arnold

Schwarzenegger, whom Chet had bested at the 1966 Mr Universe to earn his moniker of 'the Oak Slayer', had this to say.

'Chet Yorton was a legend. He beat me in the 1966 Mr. Universe when I was 19 and inspired me to be better, but he should be remembered for much more than that. He was a great father and he spread the message of health and fitness to millions. My thoughts are with his family.'

Rest easy, champ.

The Raw Egg Nationalist

REG PARK

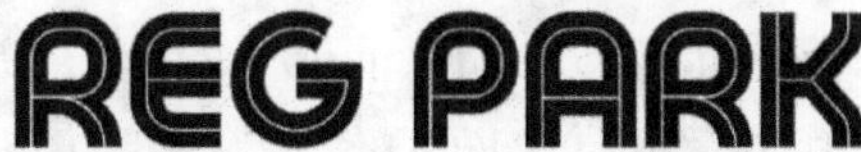

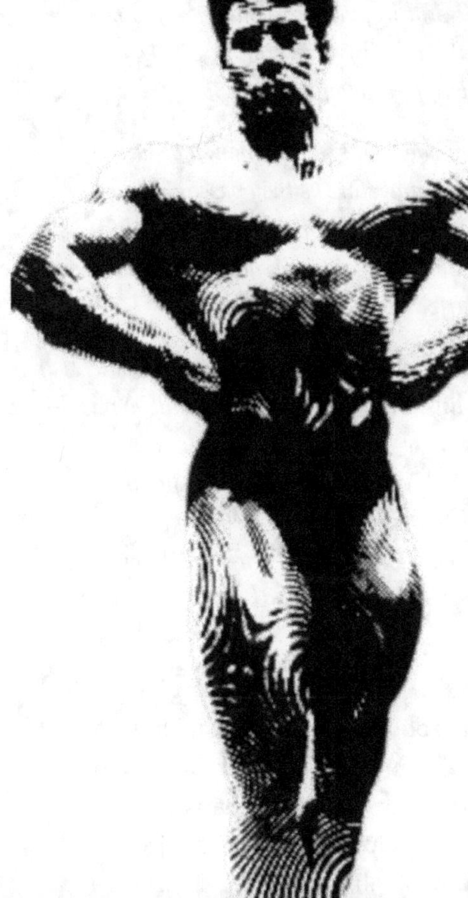

Born: 7 June 1928, Leeds England

Died: 22 November 2007, Johannesburg, South Africa

Height: 6'1"

Weight: 220lb

REG THE LEG

England, 1951. The country is still in the grip of austerity, half a decade after the massive exertions of the Second World War have come to an end. Food rationing is still in place. In London and other cities the remains of bombed-out buildings are still to be cleared. Scraggy-looking children with dirty faces play in the rubble.

Along a Camden street parades an enormous young man, a beautiful young lady on each arm. People stop and stare as they pass. He wears what must be a custom sports jacket – no tailor would stock an off-the-peg jacket with those proportions! Look at those shoulders, almost as wide as the pavement! The shutter closes. A perfect picture.

With his slick hair, chiselled jaw and winning smile, is this handsome young man a flash of California sunshine, in rainy old England? You might think so – after all that's where the world's biggest and most famous muscle men come from – but, no, this young man is not from California. He's taken the train down from Leeds, a northern city not known for its agreeable climate. This is Reg Park, England's home-grown Mr Universe.

Of the three bodybuilders in this book, Reg Park by far showed the most athletic potential as a young man; Chuck Sipes and Chet Yorton, by contrast, showed no more than average promise, and Chuck experienced disappointment and rejection in his quest to be a high-school football player. Reg's first love was also football – soccer, that is – and he played both for his local school and, by the age of 15, for Leeds United's reserve team. He was a talented gymnast and track athlete too, with an impressive time in the 100m and strong distances in the long jump and discus. He looked to be well on course for a career as a footballer when a knee injury, suffered during a game, put paid to his dream. All three bodybuilders have this in common, a transformative accident early in adulthood, but Reg's was by far the least devastating, at least physically but probably mentally too. By all rights, Chuck and Chet's lives should have ended there and then, and they returned to normal life with the kind of determination and purpose that only men who have been to the edge and back – and know it – can show.

Reg's rehabilitation was gentle. It involved wearing an iron boot – leg extension machines were unknown in England then – and progressively increasing the number of extensions. As soon as they were able to after their accidents, Chuck and Chet threw themselves into weight training, Chuck having a prior interest and Chet developing one during his convalescence; Reg's transition into bodybuilding, however, took more time. He remained more interested in gymnastics than bodybuilding. One day, though, he saw a picture of the American bodybuilder Vic Nicolette doing a lat spread in *Health and Strength* magazine, and loved what he saw, deciding that he would try to emulate the newly crowned Mr New York City; but it was not until an encounter with a local muscle man at a swimming pool that he had his first real opportunity to do so.

In the Leeds of 1946, a man like Dave Cohen stood out a country mile, with his own impressive three-of-a-kind: 17" arms, a 17" neck and 17" calves. The two young men struck up a friendship and began to train together. Their first workouts took place in Cohen's mother's front room. The room was undecorated, with no carpet, and there was only a barbell and a pair of dumbbells (guys really live in apartments like this…). Bench presses were performed laying on top of a sack on the floor, and the two men also performed overhead presses, curls, squats and pullovers. By Reg's own admission, despite his later reputation as one of the strongest bodybuilders of his time, with a 500lb bench press and 600lb squat, the weights he started lifting were small, just 40lb for presses and curls. From small acorns…

The training with Dave Cohen came to an end after just three months, when Reg had to do his two years of national service, in the army. He spent most of his time in Singapore, as a physical trainer, which involved taking soldiers in exercise sessions from nine to five each day. Although he had no access to weights during those two years, he kept himself in great shape by falling back on his gymnastics training, and his friends in Leeds kept him up to date with the world of bodybuilding by sending him copies of magazines like *Your Physique* and *Muscle Power*. The story goes that when Reg discovered the 1948 Mr Universe would be held in London, to coincide with the Olympic Games, he proclaimed that one day he was going to win the contest himself. In fact, he would be the first person to do it twice, and would win three titles overall.

Returning to England, Reg set about achieving his bold aim. He trained in his parents' back garden with a load of weights and a jerry-built rack, a wooden bench, and an improvised pulley system that ran into his bedroom from the garden. From there, he moved to a gloomy, cold rented garage, not far from his home. The building had no electricity, and in winter was lit by two candles; temperatures regularly fell below zero, but the intensity of Reg's workouts was more than enough to keep him warm. Like Chuck Sipes, who trained out of his home garage, Reg was training with neighbourhood blokes, and he also relied on a simple list of equipment that included none of the machines to be found in American or even English gyms at the time. There was a squat rack, dip bars and a chin-up bar installed in the garage, as well as lots of old plates, but nothing more than that.

His first contest was Mr Northeast Britain, in March 1949, which he won comfortably, defeating the previous year's winner. This meant an automatic invitation to that year's Mr Britain. As Chet Yorton would, Reg was blowing away the established competition with barely any training at all. An image of him in *Health and Strength* magazine from just after his victory shows him at a weight of around 205lb, with measurements as follow: neck 18″, chest 49.5″, waist 31″, upper arm 16.5″, thighs 25″ and calves 16.5″. He had only been training in the evenings after coming home from classes in business administration at a local college, but now having finished his final exams, he could up his game. With his parents' help, he became the ultimate NEET gymcel, dedicating his entire day to training, and nothing else. All the while, his parents were scrounging extra tendies – meat was still on ration in Britain until 1951 – and fixing for him. With his father's help, and with just a month before the Mr Britain competition, Reg moved to London to train at Henry Atkin's Viking Gym.

His parents' scrounging and fixing, and his own hard training, which now took place in two daily sessions, six days a week at the Viking Gym, paid off: at the end of the month in London, he was 30 pounds heavier and ready to compete for the title of Mr Britain. On the night of the contest, in the presence of John Grimek, the American bodybuilder, who had been brought over as a guest judge, Reg won, beating among others John Lees, who would go on to win the Mr Universe in 1957. 'He's a very big man!' Grimek exclaimed, noting that Reg, of all the competitors, had the most 'American' physique. Now Reg knew he really could win the Mr Universe title.

Things would not quite go to plan, however, and it would take Reg two years before he won the coveted Universe title. Between his Mr Britain victory and his first shot at the Mr Universe, in 1950, Reg travelled to America, another gift from his parents, and was able to train with many American bodybuilders, including Clarence Ross, Marvin 'the Bench-press Freak' Eder, Abe Goldberg and George Eiferman. He also met Doug Hepburn, the Olympic weightlifter, who may have taught Reg the 5x5 routine with which he has become synonymous. Hepburn would go on to be the first man in the world to bench 500lb, in 1953, and Reg would equal that feat a year later, at a *Health and Strength* show, in Bristol. When he returned to the UK to compete in the Mr Universe, Reg was ten pounds lighter from all the travelling, and this counted against him. He came second to Steve Reeves, a bodybuilder regularly cited as having one of the most, if not the most, 'aesthetic' physiques of all time. Reeves was taller and heavier than Reg, and this seemed to be the deciding factor.

> *On the day of the contest I weighed in at 215 lb. and Reeves at 225. Reeves was bigger than I was, but I was terribly muscular, with my legs, torso and arms cut up with definition. Reeves won the contest, but he was a very worried man prior to the announcement, and I recall the then editor of Health and Strength, Johnson, striving to convince him backstage that he had won. When I reflected that with less than two years' serious training I had given the very famous Steve Reeves, who had been training at least five years, such a good run for his money, I did not feel too bad, but then and there I was determined that no one would beat me in the 1951 Mr. Universe.*

Reg returned to the US, to train once more with the best bodybuilders the country had to offer. He spent a large part of his time in New York, at Abe Goldberg's gym training with Marvin Eder. His strength continued to grow, as he began to focus on 5x5 training, increasing the weight as regularly as possible. Massive strength was something Reg shared with Chuck Sipes and Chet Yorton, and through the 1950s he would continue to focus on 'power and size', rather than 'a pure bodybuilding program'; at various times and in various places he would post PRs that included a back squat of 600lb, a front squat of 405lb, a strict curl of 200lb and a 258lb one-arm dumbbell press. While in the US, he also had time to enter that year's 'America's Best Developed Athlete' contest at New York's St Nicholas Arena, which he won. Reg was now, without a doubt, a star: a phenom from across the Pond who had beaten America's best on their own soil. The rest of his training for the 1951 Mr Universe took place in South Africa. He returned to England a month before the competition, to put the finishing touches to his physique. This time, there was no doubt: Reg was even more massive than before, his competitors had no chance.

In just two years, Reg had achieved his aim; at 23 he had won the Mr Universe. Having conquered the world of bodybuilding, he turned his attention to other interests, which included a burgeoning magazine business with Joe Weider, and his own range of exercise equipment – the Reg Park Barbell Company – and supplements. Between 1951 and 1956, his training was limited by his busy schedule, which included touring the US and Hawaii, Canada, South Africa, Rhodesia and Europe. Although Reg won 'the World's Best Developed Athlete' competition while in the US, he wouldn't compete again until 1958, when he entered, and won, the Mr Universe again, becoming the first man to do so twice. By this time, he was living in South Africa with his wife, Mareon, and their two young children, and running a health centre business. He had met Mareon on an earlier trip to the country, and they had moved back and forth between Leeds and South Africa before finally settling in Johannesburg. Her brother Johnny Isaacs was also a bodybuilder, and actually placed second to Reg in the 1958 Universe.

Through the sixties, as well as continuing to train and occasionally compete – he won his third and final Mr Universe in 1965 – Reg focused on expanding his business in South Africa into a chain of health centres, all fitted out with the most modern equipment. To promote the business, he invited many bodybuilders out to South Africa to stay with him, train and put on exhibitions, including a young Arnold Schwarzenegger. Reg was already a hero to Arnold by the time they first met, at Wag Bennett's gym in east London, in 1966.

I was a 15-year-old farm kid growing up in Austria when I was first inspired by a bodybuilding magazine with a picture of him on the cover from one of his Hercules movies. My life was never the same.

Like the man who beat him to the 1950 Mr Universe title, Steve Reeves, Reg also played Hercules on the silver screen, in four Italian-made films, as well as Samson in another, between 1961 and 1965. Reg took a starstruck Arnold under his wing, and they toured the UK together before Reg invited him to come to South Africa. Arnold published an account of his stay in the German magazine *Sport Revue*. They swam on the beach at Durban, trained together and took part in various exhibitions of health and vitality. These included karate and judo performances, beauty pageants, bodybuilding competitions and individual posing routines involving Reg and Arnold.

A great experience – even for me – was Reg Park's posing freestyle, in my opinion the best in the world. Wonderful classical music accompanied his masculine, powerful poses. Nothing soft about him.

The whole experience, especially the daily three-hour training sessions with Reg, clearly had a huge effect on Arnold. The next year he won the Mr Universe for the first time, after losing the previous year to Chet Yorton. But it was not just the training that left its mark on him. The son of an austere *Sturmabteilung* and *Feldgendarmerie* officer who was awarded the Iron Cross first and second class for bravery on the Eastern Front, Arnold was not used to the love and affection Reg displayed towards his wife and children, and which he extended also to his young Austrian guest.

> *Seeing him so free with his hugs and kisses and affection, I realized that's the kind of father and husband I wanted to be. By example, he showed me what a truly full and successful life looked like.*

Reg and Arnold maintained a lifelong friendship.

The 1965 Mr Universe was Reg's last title. He competed again in the Mr Universe in 1970, but Arnold's time had come, and master now had to play second fiddle to disciple; he placed third the next year, with Bill Pearl, Chuck Sipes' mentor, winning the title; and he tried again, for the last time, and failed, in 1973.

From then until the end of his life, Reg continued to promote his businesses and the sport of bodybuilding in South Africa. In 2007, he was diagnosed with skin cancer, which eventually made it impossible for him to continue training others. One of his final public appearances was at the Arnold Classic in that year, when Arnold presented him with a lifetime achievement award. Arnold's reaction as his mentor and friend joined him onstage – barely less giddy than a simp's reaction to a DM from his favourite E-girl – and the public response in South Africa to Reg's death a few months later – both were testament to a man who had done so much to inspire others, great and not so great, to become who they truly wanted to be. Reg was blessed, too, to have children to carry on his legacy: his son Jon Jon, owner of a gym in Los Angeles, and his daughter Jeunesse, founder of a non-profit organisation dedicated to preserving the environment of the beautiful country Reg had called his home for four decades.

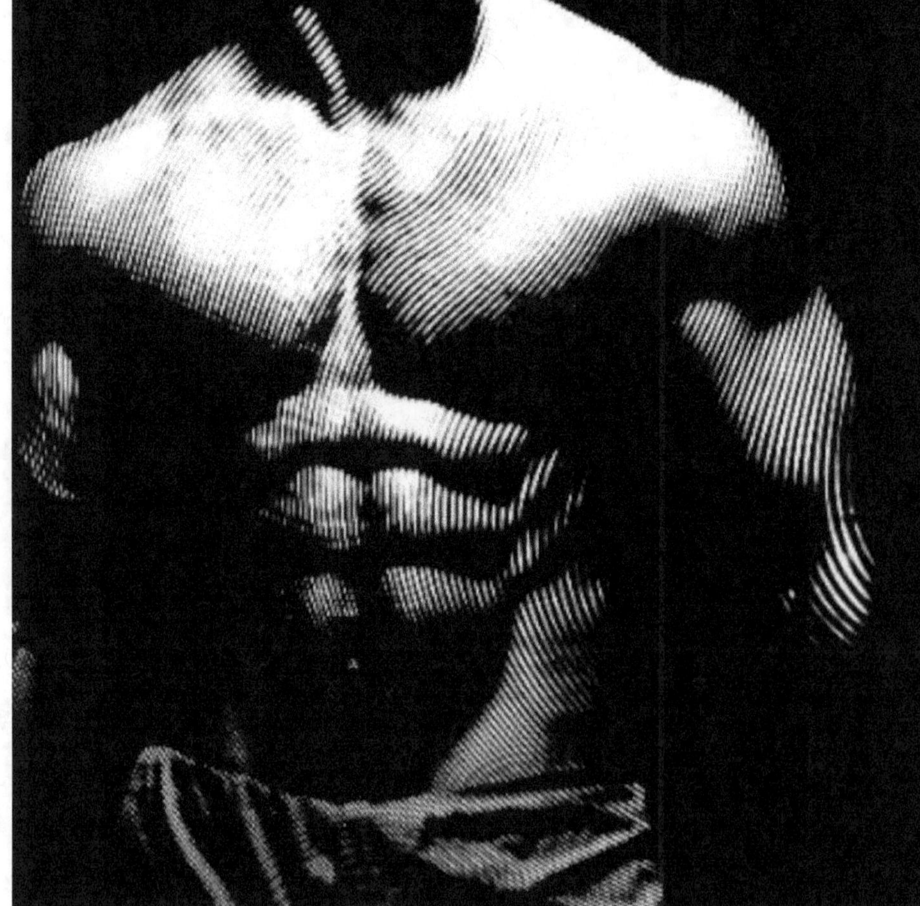
DIET AND
ROUTINE

Whatever changed over the years for Reg – like Chuck and Chet he followed what could be called an experimental approach to training – some things always remained the same: the same fundamental exercises, the same heavy weights, the same serious amounts of volume. These were the consistent principles.

The name 'Reg Park' name is synonymous with the 5x5 routine. He followed it himself at various times, and he had his students follow it too, and that would include Arnold, whose early foundations, let it not be forgotten, lay in heavy strength training, including Olympic lifts and powerlifting. Reg laid out one of the very first 5x5 routines in his pamphlet 'Strength and Bulk Training for Weight Lifters and Body Builders', published in 1960. Since then the 5x5, in which the lifter performs five sets of five reps of the main compound lifts (bench press, squat and deadlift, and sometimes other exercises including the overhead press or barbell row), has become an extremely popular training programme, especially for beginner lifters, and serves as the basis for Mark Rippetoe's Starting Strength programme and for the Stronglifts 5x5. Why 5x5? The reasoning is simple. Five reps is considered to offer a good compromise between training for strength and training for hypertrophy (muscle gain), without excessive muscular fatigue, and five sets is considered to be sufficient volume to ensure enough total stimulation. Every workout or every week, provided you manage the correct number of reps, you add more weight to the bar, and continue until you cannot do so anymore. The beginner builds strength and size at the same time, following an easy format; the progression and the results are clear, quantifiable and satisfying. The routine probably owes its origin, not to Reg, but to Mark Berry, a weightlifter of the 1930s who had his own magazine, *Strength*. Berry seems to have been the first to write, at least, about 5x5. It is possible that Reg learned of the benefits of 5x5 from the Canadian weightlifter Doug Hepburn, who won gold at the 1953 Olympics and could squat 760lb, bench 580lb and deadlift 705lb. Hepburn was training at Ed Yarick's gym in California when Reg visited in 1949.

As far as the three programmes mentioned above are concerned – Reg's 5x5, Starting Strength and Stronglifts – there are a number of similarities: the rep and set configurations, the core lifts and the number of workouts per week (three, with at least one rest day between each). In addition, Reg's 5x5 and the Starting Strength programme both involve three phases, in which the volume increases with each phase and new or different exercises are performed. There are, however, important differences. Most noticeably, Reg's 5x5 involves many more exercises than the other two programmes. Where the Starting Strength programme involves squats, bench press, deadlifts, overhead press, power cleans and chin ups, and Stronglifts involves the first four, with the addition of barbell rows, Reg's 5x5 includes all of the previous exercises, bar the chin ups and cleans, as well as hyperextensions, front squats, high pulls, calf raises, behind-the-neck presses, barbell curls and tricep extensions. Although earlier versions of the Starting Strength programme involved five sets of five reps, the most up-to-date version involves three sets of five reps, and as little as one set of five or even three reps for the deadlift per workout. Reg's 5x5, unlike the other two programmes, involves two ramp-up sets for each exercise (i.e. two lighter sets of five, then three sets of five at the day's working weight).

Despite being a precursor to both Starting Strength and Stronglifts, Reg's 5x5 actually addresses some of the most persistent criticisms of these programmes. Although Mark Rippetoe vehemently denies that assistance exercises are necessary, and claims that you should just get in the gym, do the sets then get the hell out, the lack of assistance exercises remains a bugbear of many beginners who do the programme and many established lifters who are asked to analyse it on the basis of their own experience. Starting Strength is also a lower-body-heavy routine, with up to 16 sets of primarily lower-body exercises each week (squat, deadlift and clean) as opposed to as few as nine for the upper body (bench, overhead press and chin ups); combined with Rippetoe's suggested heavy calorie intake, this can have very unfortunate physical effects. The effects of this disparity are all too visible in what is known as the 'Starting Strength body' or 'Rippetitis': massive muscular growth of the legs and arse, without corresponding growth in the upper body, which simply becomes flabby and distended. Sufferers of this troubling condition include Chloë Moretz and, if the visible symptoms are to be believed, Lana Del Rey, who appears to have taken up Starting Strength to kill time during lockdown. It's also not entirely clear that just a single set of deadlifts each workout is enough to gain the full benefits of the exercise, however taxing it may be on the nervous system. Even so, Starting Strength does have some advantages over Reg's 5x5. While the Starting Strength programme has been designed as an entry-level programme for beginners to fit in around a normal work schedule, Reg's workouts would regularly take up to three hours a day, which would probably prove unfeasible for most lifters even if they wanted to spend that much time in the gym; for beginners, such a schedule, three times a week, is likely to prove discouraging. Much is also now made, at least for the natural and not the enhanced lifter, of the supposedly dangerous increases in cortisol that very long workouts can bring. The longer a natural lifter works out, the more cortisol he releases, which jeopardises the very muscular increases he is seeking; by contrast, the enhanced lifter has enough anabolic material bouncing around his veins that long workouts and the cortisol spikes they produce are hardly a problem. Christian Thibaudeau talks a lot about this on his Youtube channel.

Reg's 5x5, as laid out in 'Strength and Bulk Training for Weight Lifters and Body Builders', is as follows. Unless otherwise indicated, the exercises are performed for five sets of five reps. Perform the exercises in the stated order.

Phase one: hyperextension (3x10), back squat, bench press, deadlift.

Phase two: hyperextension (3-4x10), front squat, back squat, bench press, overhead press, high pull, deadlift, standing barbell calf raise (5x25)

Phase three: hyperextension (4x10), front squat, back squat, overhead press, bench press, bent row, deadlift, behind-the-neck press or one-arm dumbbell press, barbell curl, lying tricep extension, standing barbell calf raise (5x25)

Each phase lasts for three months, with three workouts a week. Reg recommended resting between sets for three to five minutes during Phase One, and then reducing the rest to two minutes between sets in Phases Two and Three. As stated earlier, each set of five sets includes two lighter ramp-up sets, before three sets are completed at the day's working weight. If you complete all three working sets, increase the weight for all sets by five or ten pounds. For the hyperextensions, Reg prescribed starting with no weight on the bar at all, and then adding weight progressively with each set, while completing the specific number of reps.

This 5x5 routine is not, however, the routine that had helped him win his first major contest, Mr Britain, in 1949. Reg received the invitation to enter the contest just a month or so before it was to be held, and decided that something drastic was needed to get him into the best possible shape within that narrow window. At the Viking Gym in London, he trained in the following manner.

My life changed when I trained twice a day, six times a week. In the morning, I trained the lower body with high repetition squats, hack lifts, calf exercises and sometimes heavy bench presses. In the evening, I worked the upper body. All the squat sets were done in 20 reps with very deep breathing. The upper body work consisted of heavy standing presses, curls, bench presses, both barbell and dumbbell rows at anywhere from 6 to 10 reps per set. At this time, I did no other activity and rested whenever I was away from the weights.

Deep-breathing squats, or just breathing squats, will be returned to in depth when I talk about Chet Yorton's routine. Suffice to say that high-rep squats have been touted since the 1930s for their whole-body anabolic effects and were a staple of many a Golden Age bodybuilder's routine. Reg is said to have gained 30lb in that month of training, taking him to a competition weight of 226lb.

In South Africa, in 1966, when the young Arnold stayed with Reg, the two of them would train for up to three hours in the morning, before the heat kicked in and training would become even more hellish. Arnold wrote about their training for the German magazine *Sport Revue*. He noted that Reg preferred basic exercises like the bench press, always using 'the heaviest weights', and with only short breaks. Over the course of the three hours, 100 sets would be completed, including 20 sets for the calves, which Reg trained every day.

When it came to eating, given his size Reg probably ate even more than Chuck or Chet. Bucketloads. A truckful of food. 'Like a king', in his own words.

I liked to eat like a king, but only food that was good for me. I ate prodigious amounts of food during the day, but adhered to a very balanced diet with everything in proper proportions.

> *My favorite food is steak, which I sometimes eat twice a day. I also like salads, orange juice and wine. I have a wine cellar in my home. I also have used protein supplements and take vitamin and mineral tablets.*

But Earle Liedeman, of *Iron Man* magazine, tells a slightly different story.

> *Once, when dining with Reg, he gargled three large plates of vegetable soup, then gulped chunks from his extra large and thick steak without his teeth sinking into the meat once, apparently, next stuffed many side dishes of vegetables into his ever open mouth and these include an extra large pair of baked potatoes, a huge bowl of salad, three glasses of milk and the last, the piece de resistance, a big dish of ice cream with cake. And all this, mind you, in about ten minutes. Gee! I've seen hungry bloodhounds gobble down food, but Reg Park wins a can of fried grasshoppers as second place for amount, and first place for speed.*

In his 1954 article, 'An Everyday Diet for the Bodybuilder', Reg noted that 'the majority of musclemen seem to have a very sweet tooth so if you are not troubled with being overweight, by all means indulge – but home made cakes are best'; the author, clearly, was a typical muscle man in that regard, at least. Both Chuck and Chet, by contrast, swore off any kind of white-flour products and almost all sweet foods, and Chet almost entirely swore off carbohydrates altogether; although he wasn't above cheating when circumstances dictated, especially when he was travelling to and from shows. Quantity, quantity, quantity was a key Reg Park principle, one he advocated for others.

> *I have seen youngsters desirous of putting on weight, drinking lemon tea and eating Ryvita when they should have been drinking milk and eating brown bread and butter with plenty of honey on it.*

Of the three bodybuilders featured in this book, Reg was probably the least discerning in his eating habits. Still, by comparison with what that might mean today – the endless shovelling of vegetable-oil and GMO corn-syrup zog snacks – there can be no doubt that 'quality' was also an important principle for him. His diet was based on the same natural protein and fat sources that Chuck and Chet consumed when they were training: lots of milk, lots of eggs, lots of red meat. Reg drank up to two gallons of milk a day, and ate at least a dozen eggs; by some accounts he ate as much as eight pounds of steak a day, a feat which would only have been possible if, as Liedeman says, he swallowed the meat without chewing. He was not, apparently, a fan of raw eggs, but preferred them cooked, believing them to be healthier.

Besides his fondness for home-made cakes, Reg had other idiosyncrasies. During his time in South Africa, Arnold remembered that Reg would have a 5am meal of cornflakes sprinkled with milk and protein powder. He also insisted on sipping orange juice between his daily 100 sets – so he drank quite a volume presumably; he had been doing this since the late 1940s, when he would drink 'two pints of diluted concentrated orange juice with glucose and honey mixed in it at every workout'.

One thing Reg and Chet definitely had in common was alcohol consumption. Where Chet favoured beer and whiskey, Reg preferred wine and stout, especially Guinness, when he was training to put on weight. Guinness is colloquially known as a 'meal in a glass', but despite the feeling of extreme satiety it brings – I've never been able to manage more than about two pints of it without wanting to take a nap – it actually contains fewer calories than your average pint of lager. The much-vaunted mineral content of Guinness also appears to be a myth. I say more about alcohol in Chet's 'Routine and Diet' section.

CHUCK SIPES

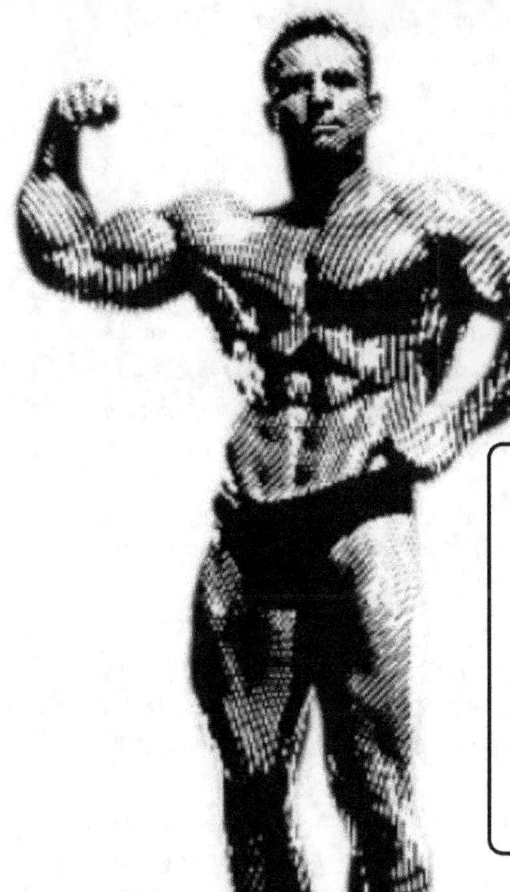

Born: 22 August 1932,
Sterling, Illinois

Died: 24 February 1993,
Siskiyou County,
California

Height: 5'9"

Weight: 220lb

THE IRON KNIGHT

For a week now they have followed him, climbing further into the mountains. From time to time they stop, and he points out to the young men some species of tree or plant, a bird of prey high above, circling in the cloudless sky – even a mountain lion across the valley beyond. They look at these things, but observe with just as much wonder the enormous musculature of the man's outstretched arms and shoulders; and when he walks in front of them, the vast spread of his back, the neck that seems to have been transplanted from some mythical creature, and his calves, like two thick joints of ham, above the ankle socks and boots. They have seen men like this before, but never outside the pages of a comic book. In the afternoons, when the sun is less intense, they find a shaded spot, drop their packs and exercise together. When night comes, they sleep soundly under a canopy of stars none of them have ever seen back in the city.

Now, in the evenings, after supper, under his guidance their talk moves from the usual chit-chat, jokes and things young men talk about to a more serious topic: how each of them has come to find himself on the wrong side of the law. At first, the young men have trouble opening up. It's not easy to talk like this. Nobody has ever listened to them before. Their thoughts and feelings have never mattered. But this seems to be his real superpower: he shows them that they do matter. They are not just victims of circumstance, the ever-present criminal element of society, but masters of their own destiny. They have a choice. When they return home in three weeks' time, each of them will be determined to be a better man – to be just like Chuck Sipes.

An Illinoisian by birth, Chuck Sipes moved to Modesto, California with his family as a child. Although he had already been introduced to weight training as a scrawny wannabe high-school football player, Chuck had his real introduction to bodybuilding only after a taste of high-speed dirt that would have killed anybody other than a man destined to be a demigod; so too Chet Yorton, whose accident was arguably worse. Before their respective dates with near-death, neither man had displayed much evidence of the physical prowess with which his name would later be synonymous. During his early days as a schoolboy lifter, under the tutelage of his neighbour Chuck Coker, Sipes showed no real interest in bodybuilding at all.

Chuck began his competitive bodybuilding career unwillingly. Chuck Coker recalls that when Sipes was a lifting competitor in his junior college days in Modesto, there was one occasion when a physique contest was held in connection with the lifting. Chuck's buddies on the team filled out an entry form to the physique contest, then informed Chuck that he had to get up on stage and pose. He said no at first, but then did sort of a stroll across the stage and hit a few poses.

(This may be the first recorded instance of the Chad stride.) Throughout his bodybuilding career, the posing, rather than the lifting, would remain the part that least interested Chuck, and his lack of a polished posing routine probably cost him a number of titles he would otherwise have won.

After graduating from school, Chuck decided to become a paratrooper, joining the US Army's famous 82nd Airborne. He served for three years until during a practice jump his parachute failed and he became entangled with another trooper, falling 70 feet to the ground. (Some have suggested that the impact may have been the cause of the mysterious and hugely destructive Tunguska Event; however plausible the claim that the earth would come off a distant second to Chuck Sipes in a collision, the disparity of dates and locations is enough to disprove this.) Chuck spent the next four months in hospital, recovering from serious head injuries that would leave their mark in the longer term with epilepsy and severe depression; tragically, the depression would dog him for the rest of his life, and was almost certainly a contributor to his death by suicide, in 1993.

But our story continues in 1952. After his time in hospital, Chuck began to receive disability pay for his injuries, until a visit to a military doctor brought those payments to an end: how could a man with a body like that be *disabled*? The work with Chuck Coker, and the hard paratrooper's training, had clearly already provided him with the basis for his later marvellous physique. Chuck now returned to California and normal life (if by 'normal' you mean the life of a lumberjack) with the intention of becoming a bodybuilder; and not just any bodybuilder but the best in the world. He sought out Bill Pearl, who won his first Mr Universe competition the next year, in London, beating, among others, a 23-year-old Scot by the name of Sean Connery. Pearl would win the Universe title an unheralded four times before his retirement in 1971, and receive the moniker of the 'World's Best-built Man of the Century'; he has been described as 'Arnold, before there was Arnold', and 'bodybuilding's first true crossover superstar', both of which could also just as equally be applied to Reg Park as well. For Chuck, the mould was set: not only was Pearl possessed of a beautiful physique, but he was also extremely strong. He regularly dressed up in the garb of a Sandow-era strongman – replete with leotard or fig leaf, fake moustache and period backdrop – and performed feats of strength like bending spike nails and blowing up hot water bottles until they exploded; he could also bench press 500lb, at a time when very few men could. Chuck would go on to perform similar feats in similarly absurd getups, bending steel rebars held between his teeth, ripping phonebooks in half with his bare hands or crushing spike nails, just like his mentor. His mentor's bench press PR he would beat by a full hundred pounds. While Chuck was competing, the only man stronger at benching – in the world – was Pat Casey, who was also 135lb heavier than him.

After around five years of training, in 1958 Chuck won his first competition, in California, the Amateur Athletic Union's Mr North California contest; he was 26. He also placed in the top ten that year in a number of other regional and national contests, including the AAU's Junior Mr America and Mr America contests. In 1959, Chuck would get his first taste of real success, winning the IFBB Mr America, before winning the 1960 Mr Universe. In the mid-sixties, he turned his attention to the Mr Olympia contest for the first time. In the 1966 Olympia, won by Larry Scott, he placed third, and the following year, he came second to Sergio Oliva; along with Chet Yorton and Frank Zane, Oliva, a Cuban bodybuilder often referred to as 'the Myth', was one of only three people ever to beat Arnold in competition. Chuck continued to compete to the end of the decade and into the early seventies. After his close failures at the 1966 and 1967 Olympias, he won the NABBA World Championship in 1967 and Mr California and Mr World in 1968. In 1970, he came second in the medium class of the Mr Universe, whose overall class was won by Arnold. Chuck finally retired from competition in 1974 following his win in the over-40s category of the Mr Pacific Coast.

The intensity not just of Chuck's competition training but of his life in general was legendary. Where most would struggle to fit a bodybuilding routine in around any kind of full-time job, Chuck, being Chuck, managed to work out after full days chopping trees as a lumberjack or in sawmills up and down the Pacific Coast. He credited his massive 18" forearms to this hard work, at a time when many bodybuilders did little or no separate forearm training; he considered his forearms to be essential to his massive strength. And it was no mere routine he performed after putting down his chainsaw and hardhat and washing the dirt, sweat and sawdust from his skin. In the run-up to the 1968 Mr World, for instance, Chuck was training every body part three days a week, working up to his maximum lifts every other day and using all sorts of high-intensity schemes, such as the 1-10/10-1. As well as lifting heavy often, Sipes believed in maximising intensity, reducing his rest times between sets to as little as ten seconds. More on his training anon, anon.

This rugged lifestyle, while hardening his muscles superbly, did nothing to harden Chuck's heart. Said Dave Draper of Chuck:

This man, who looked like a pile of rocks and lifted steel like a crane and shredded and crumpled anything he got his hands on, was a gentleman, a peacemaker and an artist. He insisted you go first while he carried your load; he counseled troubled young men in the California state penal system and created with brush and oils on large canvas incredible old west paintings in marvelous detail. Chuck Sipes was a mighty good man.

The term 'muscular Christian' could have been coined, in the most literal sense, to describe Chuck; and I can think of few who would be better placed to lead a revival of that much maligned and misunderstood doctrine than the Iron Knight himself. Before and after retiring from competitive bodybuilding, he spent 20 years coaching and mentoring troubled inner-city youths for the California Youth Authority. Chuck put his love and knowledge of the California wilderness to good use by leading groups of young men on three-week expeditions into the forest. There, after the initial bewilderment had passed, he would help them to speak about and understand the difficulties of their lives. These campfire conversations became the basis of many lifelong friendships between Chuck and his mentees, who would continue to visit him through the years. The expeditions also involved impromptu workouts in which cables would be wrapped around trees and various exercises were performed. The success rate of Chuck's work was overwhelming: according to the superintendent of Folsom Prison, 96% of the youths Chuck mentored did not return to jail. Ever humble, Chuck said,

> *One of my objectives was to win the kids over to Christianity, and introduce them to a more positive way of life. It may not have been the answer for all, but it was a start in the right direction.*

The use of drugs was one of Chuck's particular concerns. A heartfelt letter about your high school's drug problem would almost invariably guarantee an appearance from the man himself, who would turn up, put on an awesome exhibition of strength and then give a stirring speech on the virtues of clean living and exercise. It was drugs, in particular, that led to Chuck's departure from competitive bodybuilding, in the early 1970s. A few years after Chet Yorton was turned on to the dangers of steroids,

> *Chuck was rooming with another world famous bodybuilder overseas during a posing exhibition. Chuck walked into their hotel room and found the other bodybuilder with a needle in his butt. Chuck asked what was going on and was told, "Oh, you have to do this to compete these days."*

Chuck, however, disagreed, and began to speak out against steroid use. 'CHARLTON HESTON'S MUSCULAR DOUBLE' featured on the cover of the February 1971 issue of *Muscle Training* magazine, beside the caption: 'MR AMERICA CHUCK SIPES SAYS: DRUGS ARE DESTROYING MUSCLE MEN'. Chuck effectively retired from bodybuilding after the article was published; although he competed one final time in 1974. Of course, he continued to train, and remained in amazing shape. Part of his community work involved acting as the weight trainer at a youth facility, and a fellow employee remembers how when Chuck was in his mid-fifties, with grey shoulder-length hair, 'this O.G. was still cut up, I couldn't believe someone at this age could continue to stay in shape'. Chuck also continued trekking in the wilderness, which became the subject of another of his hobbies: painting. While it's hard to find pictures of Chuck's paintings on the internet, one image can be found of Chuck posing proudly next to a fantastically detailed mountain river scene, with two riders in the foreground. The date of the painting isn't clear, but Chuck has grey in his beard and his hair is receding; yet the famous physique is still evident – the enormous forearms and biceps, especially.

During the later years of Chuck's life, his mood darkened, and nothing his family and friends could do could change it; life seemed to hold him with a weaker and weaker grip. His painting no longer brought the same satisfaction, and bureaucracy began to get in the way of the expeditions that had done such good for the deprived young men of California. Ultimately, the reason why a man like Chuck Sipes would take his own life – simple brain chemistry or something far less simple – must remain a mystery. Joe Roark, of the Roark Report, puts it well:

What causes a man, who cheers up everyone, to change so that he cannot be cheered up by those he loves? Big Chuck was becoming little Chuck inside himself. A man whose family loved him, whose artwork was respected, whose cell-mates (so to speak) became sell-mates and are forever in his debt, whose stupendous strength and physique accomplishments were no longer able to re-kindle his former bright attitudes.

Chuck was buried in his buckskins, a mountain man to the last. One of the many young men whose life Chuck had helped to transform read the eulogy. 'CHUCK SIPES – MEETS THE SUN', his gravestone reads: back into the light he had shone on all those who knew him.

DIET AND ROUTINE

Chuck followed what could be described as an instinctual approach to both his routine and his diet. Rather than sticking to any one approach rigidly, he would pay close attention to his body and how he felt, and make changes accordingly. Nevertheless, he did follow certain principles, which included lifting heavy more or less all the time (right up to his maximum lifts), minimising rest between sets and using other intensification schemes. He appears to have favoured two-day splits which resulted in him working every body part three times a week. There is a lot of information available about various different programmes and routines Chuck followed or is said to have followed, including the pamphlets Chuck himself wrote; Chuck was very keen to document his routines, especially after coming out against steroid use in bodybuilding. I haven't tried to be comprehensive here, but have reproduced a small selection of what I have found; included are his bench press specialisation routine, including separate tricep work, and some notes on how he developed his famous forearms, as well as some of his intensification routines.

Although Chuck initially trained with Bill Pearl, later he moved to training at home. This is essentially what Reg Park did, but in reverse. Chuck had few training partners, and those he had were local neighbourhood blokes, not the superstars to be found at Pearl's gym, Vince Gironda's gym or the original Gold's Gym. Norm Komich, the young mentee who read the eulogy at Chuck's funeral, remembers his surprise at finally visiting the place where Chuck had trained for his 1968 Mr World win.

We were very anxious to see the famous home gym of Chuck and we headed for the garage. I cannot tell you the shock we experienced when we saw the basic and actually crude setup he had. The primary piece was a wooden power rack.

Chuck didn't have an Olympic bar, and when he needed some extra weight for his heavy 'support' movements, discussed below, he went to the local train yard and took some old train wheels. He had no machines or squat rack – not even a dumbbell rack. The only other piece of 'equipment' he had was some nylon straps set into the rafters, so that he could do wide hangs to stretch his lats. The lesson for gymbros everywhere should be clear, and is all the more vital at this present moment, when commercial gyms could close at any time.

One aspect of Chuck's routine that has been vindicated many times over is his insistence on generally beginning his workouts with heavy (power)lifting, and then following it with bodybuilding exercises. Since Chuck's time, this approach has been used to great effect by stacked power-builders like Roger Estep, who helped explode the myth that powerlifters have to be monstrously fat. Variously described as 'the best built man in powerlifting' (*Powerlifting USA*, June 1980) and 'the bastard child of Gaetan Dugas and the Incredible Hulk' (me, now), Estep combined a powerlifting total of well over 2 000lb at 198lb, with a physique that would not have been out of place next to Mike Mentzer on the Mr Olympia stage. After beginning his routine with heavy squats and bench press, or squats and deadlifts, and various power assistance exercises like high or low box squats, Estep would always finish with bodybuilding exercises. Look at Joe Ladnier, Kirk Karkowski or Bobby Myers for further examples.

Chuck's bench press specialisation routine involved working up to a maximum bench press and then doing sets of partial reps at various heights from the chest. Start by doing two warmup sets of 8, then do two sets with a weight you can manage for 6 reps with good form; the weight should be heavy, but not so heavy that you struggle to complete the sets. Now increase the weight and drop to two sets of 4 reps, and again for two sets of 2. Finally, aim to hit your max, and then try another single, or even two. Repeat the process lifting the bar from pins set at the middle of the range of motion (6,6,4,4,2,2), then again with the pins set further up (4,4,2,2), and then finally with the pins set about an inch from lockout. It's not clear how many reps he advocated doing in this final position, which he called a 'support position'; since he believed in the importance of acclimatising yourself to heavier weights than you are capable of lifting fully, he probably increased the weight beyond his max for a conventional bench press. I can testify to the value of loading the bar for a squat with a weight that is well in excess of your max, and then stepping out and just holding the weight on your back for a minute or longer, before walking it back in; this builds a sense of confidence as well as preparing the muscles for lifting heavier loads down the line. The Snakepham Youtube Channel has many videos of Chinese Olympic weightlifters doing this regularly as part of their training. Try it.

To improve the bench press, Chuck also recommended focusing on developing the triceps. He considered this to be among the most important accessory work you could do for the bench. In his pamphlet 'Triceps Power', he notes how weightlifters looking to improve their bench press had neglected the triceps, thinking that extra shoulder work and then pectoral work would pay off most, before realising, by process of elimination, that in fact it must be the triceps they should be working on.

> *At first, no one could say for sure. Maybe it was the delts. So they tried military presses. They didn't prove to help the bench a great deal. So they tried parallel dips with plenty of weight. Pat Casey did them endlessly, dropping to an extremely low position, but they ground up his shoulders, and he stopped. Extreme range of motion like the military and dip was out; the pecs and delts were out. That left the triceps.*

The two exercises he favoured for triceps were the cheat pullover and the rack lockout. Cheat pullovers can either be performed off the bench, as Bill West did, or with the weight on the floor, in the manner of Pat Casey. Bill West put a towel on the bench and then bounced the weight off it, allowing him to lift heavier weights. Casey, by contrast, placed the barbell on the floor at the end of the bench, with his feet hooked on the supports. The movement off the floor is more like a bent-arm pullover, which then transitions into an extension at the end of the movement. For the rack lockout, sit on a 60° incline bench in a power rack. Take a 6-inch grip on the bar and do short skull crushers to lockout, keeping your upper arm vertical.

Chuck created his own variation of the wrist curl, which, along with the copious axe-work he did, helped to grow his massive forearms. Take a dumbbell in your hand, sit and lay the top of your forearm on your thigh, allowing the hand with the dumbbell to hang over the knee; now twist your torso so that the elbow of the dumbbell arm is under the opposite armpit. Wrist curl the weight from that position. Other exercises Chuck performed included reverse curls, rubber ball squeezes and roller exercises, either with a newspaper (rolling the newspaper up as tightly as possible and then unrolling it) or with a rolling device such as the one I described making on my Twitter timeline.

I've already said that Chuck would try to minimise rest between sets as much as possible, sometimes to as little as ten seconds. Another intensification method he used was pyramid sets, in particular the 1-10/10-1. The method is simple: you do one rep, rest for a short period of time, then two reps, rest again and so on, all the way up to ten, and then back down to one. Keep the rest to an absolute minimum. If you can manage the full scheme of ten, you've done 100 reps. If you fail going up, descend from there. This scheme can be used for any exercise, and is very effective as a burner to finish working a particular body part; for instance, after three sets of heavy cheat curls, do a 1-10/10-1 with much less weight on the bar for an awesome pump.

Like his gym setup, Chuck's diet was simple; although, again, he did experiment and try some interesting things. He gave the following advice:

Eat a well-balanced diet of meats, fish, fruits and vegetables. Avoid high-calorie foods such as bread, cake, candy, macaroni products and all foods containing white flour and white sugar. High-calorie foods add fat to your waistline and will make your abdominal training a whole lot tougher than it should be.

This is not at all dissimilar from the diet Chet Yorton followed; although it should be noted that Chuck does not appear to have run as close to a ketogenic diet as Chet did (but see the end of this section for a note on fasting). Apart from on rare occasions when a virtue had to be made of necessity, Chet consumed no bread or other starches at all. What carbohydrates he did consume almost all came from the copious volumes of raw milk he drank. By contrast, Chuck would eat brown rice, wholemeal bread and cereals regularly.

Chuck gave the eminently sensible recommendation that your food consumption should mirror your activity levels. Given that Chuck worked as a lumberjack, as well as performing hard and heavy workouts that would have the average gymbro crying into their Gold's Gym gloves, he generally appears to have eaten a lot of food. It's not easy to find a definitive daily diet, and given the openness with which approached his lifting regime, listening to his body and making alterations whenever he felt they were appropriate, it's probable that he made many changes to his diet, as suited him.

In his 'Nutritional Plan for Strength and Power' pamphlet, Chuck advocates the following diet, including frequent meals (up to a total of six) and a variety of supplements.

Breakfast: A glass of fruit juice, whole grain cereal, wholewheat bread and honey, and a protein drink (2 glasses of milk, 2 raw eggs, protein powder and flavouring), with supplements (1 vitamin C table), 1tsp wheat germ oil, 1 vitamin and mineral capsule, 1 B12 tablet and a handful of liver tablets

Mid-morning: protein drink (as before) and a handful of nuts

Lunch: 2 sandwiches (cheese, meat or peanut butter), fresh green salad, 2 glasses of milk, either a thick soup or cottage cheese, either jello or a pudding, and 1tsp of wheat germ oil

Mid-afternoon: protein drink (as before) and fresh fruit

Dinner: meat (broiled or baked), fresh green salad, vegetables, 2 glasses of milk, ice cream or fruit salad and 1 vitamin C tablet

Bedtime: protein drink (as before)

Chuck particularly recommended adding 'germ oils, sunflower seeds, papaya, peanuts and lots of milk' to your regular diet. Most of us raw egg nationalists, Twitter frogs and RWBBs would instantly run screaming at the suggestion of adding PUFAs (polyunsaturated fatty acids (i.e. germ oils)) to our diets, rather than subtracting them, because of what we know about the appalling health effects they've had since their introduction as alternative 'healthy' fats, beginning in the mid-twentieth century. This is a strong contender for the most disgraceful of many disgraceful scams spun by the Lords of Lies on the subject of nutrition: imagine convincing people to pay to eat paint thinners instead of the healthy animal fats we've been eating since the dawn of time! Ray Peat talks extensively about this truly Satanic plot – about how industrial products came to be used to fatten first pigs and then humans – and if you haven't read what he has to say, you should – NOW.[1] As I mention with Chet Yorton and his beer and soy powder, these things don't seem to have done Chuck any harm; but then we've been gutthexxed and poisoned to a degree that far outstrips what our grandparents or even our parents had to endure. Eternal vigilance is the price of freedom from the tyranny of zogriculture.

The other suggestions are hard to disagree with, though. Assuming the nuts and seeds are fresh, raw and not roasted, you'll be fine (roasting, among other effects, reduces the antioxidant content and also oxidises the fats, which is bad news for your body). Papain, an enzyme, is a magical ingredient of papaya that makes it a highly beneficial addition

---

[1] Most of these essays are available at raypeat.com. A good start would be the essay 'Unsaturated vegetable oils: toxic'.

to your diet. The enzyme aids in the digestion of protein –
essential if you are on a high-protein diet – and also helps to
clear the intestinal walls. Many bodybuilders eat lots of
pineapple for a similar reason. I generally have a dessert of
pineapple and sheep's milk yoghurt after my evening meal.
Finally milk, and by that Chuck meant raw milk, should be a
sine qua non for the bodybuilder of Indo-European descent.
'Muh lactose intolerant' – sorry, but it's unlikely: what you're
probably intolerant of is the carageenan, a seaweed-derived
zogchem that is used to homogenise supermarket milk;
another use is causing tumours and various inflammatory
conditions in lab mice… Rarely can I resist the opportunity to
cite the Mongols and other pastoral peoples, such as the
Yamnaya, as evidence for why milk consumption is a good
thing; just look at what they did and what they thought of the
settled agricultural peoples they conquered.[2] (I'm sure you've
seen the widely circulated image of the three Mongolian
wrestlers, and of course you know the Chad Pastoralist meme.)
I've already mentioned Reg Park's massive milk consumption
– two gallons a day – and Chet also seems to have consumed a
similar amount. In the section on Chet's routine and diet, I
mention the 'squats and milk' diet, which was responsible for
the sudden massive growth of many an old-school lifter.

As well as the earlier recipe for a protein shake, Chuck also
liked to use the following recipe, which makes a delicious ice
cream (see my Twitter page); as ice cream, this could fit nicely

---

[2] Read J. Weatherford, *Genghis Khan and the Making of the Modern World* (New
York, 2004).

into the 'Diet for Strength and Power' routine outlined above as part of dinner.

- 300ml milk
- A scoop of protein powder
- 2 spoonfuls of blackstrap molasses
- 1 spoonful of honey
- 1 spoonful of Ovaltine
- 1 banana
- 1 scoop of ice cream

Chuck consumed no refined sugars as part of his diet, preferring honey and blackstrap molasses to sweeten his shakes and provide carbohydrates. The benefits of blackstrap molasses deserve some comment. Blackstrap is a by-product of refining cane sugar. First, the cane is mashed, producing juice, which is then boiled and reduced to produce cane syrup. A further boiling produces molasses, and yet another produces blackstrap, which is thick and tangy and has a lower sugar content than standard molasses. Blackstrap contains a variety of minerals and vitamins, including iron, calcium, magnesium, B6 and selenium. Magnesium, in particular, is a mineral that many people are deficient in. Its importance cannot be overstated: it is essential to enzyme function, protein synthesis, muscle and nerve function, blood glucose and blood pressure regulation, and D3 formation. With low magnesium levels, individuals, especially in northern climes, are liable to Seasonal Affective Disorder, sluggishness, loss of appetite, nausea and vomiting, as well as a compromised immune system. For further information on magnesium supplementation, look no further than Grimm's Apothecary (@Grimhood); just don't take it personally if he blocks you. If you're worried about the iron levels, consume blackstrap with milk: the calcium strongly inhibits iron uptake. This is one of the reasons why it is a good idea to consume animal blood in ice cream form. Yes, really: look up my recipe for sanguinaccio dolce ice cream, on Twitter.

In an interview from just after his final competition, the 1974 Mr Pacific Coast, Chuck described some experiments he had conducted with fasting. His interest in the subject may have derived from his experiences in the wilderness, when he wouldn't have been able to maintain his normal diet. After spending a month outdoors, Chuck might lose as much as 15 or 20lb of weight, but his friends marvelled at the way he could regain that lost weight simply by eating more and lifting.

Do you remember that two week fast that I went on last summer? Well, I did a little experiment... During this time I took in no food, all I had each day was fresh vegetable broth once a day, and fresh fruit juice mixed in water twice a day. During this time I was working out with weights, running, and swimming. The first five days I felt rather weak and had a few periods of depression.

But then after the fifth day something strange happened. All of a sudden I started feeling stronger than I had previously, yet I was still taking in no food. What happens is that your body starts living off of old dead cells and once you are rid of these cells your body starts to function with greater efficiency.

What Chuck is clearly describing is autophagy, one of the most highly touted benefits of fasting, especially intermittent fasting, which has become a big trend in the health and fitness world these days. The theory is simple: the term literally means 'self-eating', as the body rejuvenates itself by consuming and replacing damaged cell components. My friend Jawbrah (@Zyzzrespecter) has posted some good information on this subject.

At this time, Chuck had also decided to cut down on his meat consumption, jokingly referring to himself as a vegetarian, while admitting that he still consumed fish and white meat. He had decided it would be unhealthy for him, past 40, to continue carrying his competition weight of 225lb, so he had slimmed down to around 195lb. He said he had cut his meals down to two a day, sometimes skipping lunch. Asked what he would do if he wanted to gain the weight back, he said that he would increase the weight he was lifting and then

I would also start drinking some raw milk and increase my food intake, but I would still eat only the natural foods that I eat now.

You know — fruits, vegetables, honey, whole wheat bread, granola, rose hip tea, chicken and fish. I believe that there is great value in fish, whereas the value of meat is not that great.

CHET YORTON

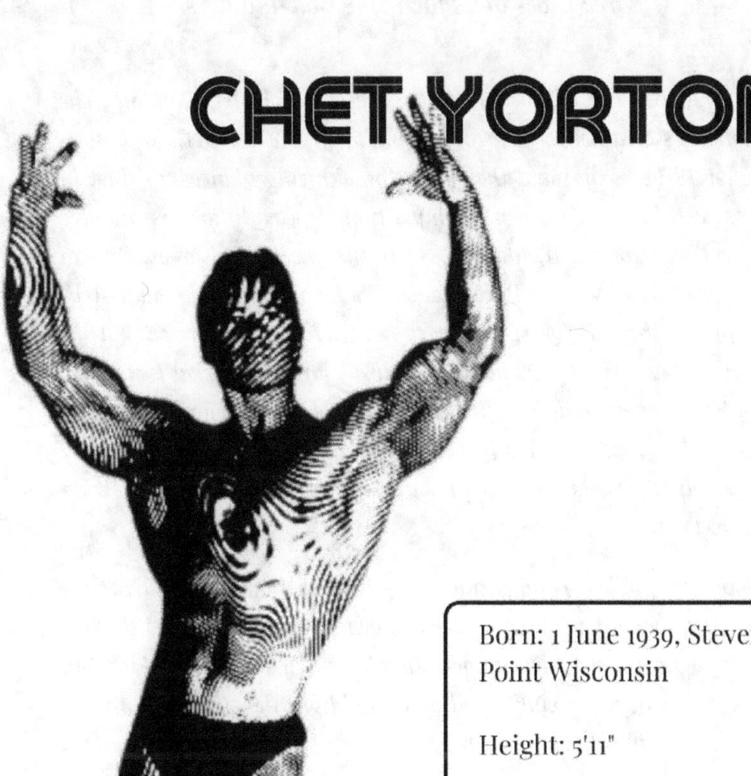

Born: 1 June 1939, Stevens Point Wisconsin

Height: 5'11"

Weight: 220lb

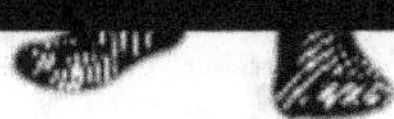

The NABBA Mr Universe 1966. The Royal Hotel, London. The Austrian's confidence is at an all-time high. He is Mr Europe now, at just 19 years old, and the subject of admiring glances not just in the street, but also from his competition, especially for his massive 20" arms. Confident, that is, until he meets the favourite, an American from Malibu Beach called Chet Yorton. As the man steps out of the lift, the Austrian's heart sinks. He knows at once that the magazines are right: this man will win. A formality. Chet is not just big: he's tanned, defined, with every muscle separate and crossed by veins like a roadmap. He has a look of athleticism and energy, the ready suppleness of an apex predator. By comparison, the Austrian just feels fat.

Despite the applause and enthusiasm of the small audience during the first day, when the contest is decided behind closed doors, as the two men line up directly next to each other before the judges, the Austrian knows that their proximity will only highlight the superiority of the other man's physique.

At the Victoria Palace Theatre the next night, during the public performance, the Austrian is pushed back on stage for an encore. The crowd love him. Perhaps he really could do this! But then Chet Yorton takes to the stage for his posing routine. Taut, powerful, determined, he explodes from one pose to the next like a machine. He knows all sorts of little tricks to make his muscles pop out, to make his waist look smaller or display multiple muscles at once. 'I am the winner,' his face says – and he is right.

The young Austrian will never experience such humiliation again; though he takes it graciously, like a man. He will study every aspect of the science of bodybuilding in the closest detail. He will become a legend: Arnold, the 'Austrian Oak'. And Chet will always be known as the 'Oak Slayer', one of just three men to take him on in competition and win.

*

I lay in the car for half an hour until the police arrived and pried the doors open with crowbars to release me. The ambulance rushed me to the St. Francis hospital where the doctors then debated about amputating my right leg, but [with my] not consenting, they then performed surgery on it for four and one-half hours, putting in a five-inch steel plate and eight screws around my right thigh bone. Three days later they performed surgery on my left thigh bone and at which time they inserted a stainless steel rod about an inch in diameter, inside the femur bone of my left leg from the hip to knee by cutting my hip open and drilling out the hollow where the rod was to be inserted down the center of the thigh bone.

The teenage Chet Yorton had just survived a devastating car crash. He was alive, but things could scarcely have been said to be looking up for him. His body, like the car he had been a passenger in, was wrecked. As the car left the road and hit a tree, the impact of bracing himself against the floor had driven his hips from their sockets; his thighs were shattered, his left arm lacerated deeply from elbow to wrist. Miraculously, the piece of windshield glass that had pierced his left eyeball had stopped an eighth of an inch from penetrating his brain – an injury that would almost certainly have killed him. Instead, he suffered only a concussion. At this point, a future as a physique champion could barely have seemed less probable; he would be lucky if he even walked again, let alone got up on stage to pose majestically to the theme from 'Exodus'.

After surgery, with his lower body totally encased, Chet lay in traction for a month. Physical therapy began when the cast was removed from his left leg. Once he could bend his left leg enough, he was allowed to use crutches, placing his bodyweight on his right leg, which remained in cast. But his misfortune continued as soon as he returned home. Losing his balance on the porch, he fell down the front steps, re-breaking his left leg. Further surgery was required, and he would spend the next four months in a wheelchair; he would have to re-learn how to walk on crutches.

It's from this point that his story becomes almost laughably improbable. Within just two years of his brush with death, Chet would be competing in physique competitions – *and winning*; from physical wreck to physical specimen, in just 24 months. The story goes that it was while convalescing in his wheelchair at the hospital that he saw a pair of dumbbells and decided to start pumping iron, for the very first time. Whatever athletic potential the young Chet had, it had not been much in evidence during his teenage years, when he had been an unremarkable sportsman; fast forward seven months from his first encounter with a dumbbell and he had put on 55lb of solid mass. His spectacular gains continued, and within a year and a half he had reached a massive 240lb (at 5' 11", remember), at which point he began to cut, down to a more svelte 210lb in readiness for his first competition. Of course, he won.

The refinement, and with it the victories, continued. He won titles at regional and national level through the 1960s, and began to appear on the covers of various magazines, including *Strength and Health* (1964), *Mr America* (1965), *Muscle Builder* (1965 and 1967) and *Iron Man* (1967). It was at 26, around eight years after he first began training, that Chet won the 1966 amateur Mr Universe (tall division), in London, the victory that earned him the moniker 'the Oak Slayer'. At that time, Arnold was already on his way to becoming the most famous bodybuilder in the world, having been crowned Mr Europe at 19; but in his own words, he looked like 'uncooked bread dough' on stage next to Yorton. Yorton had the modern bodybuilder's three most-prized attributes in spades – size, definition and vascularity; Arnold, who had only size, was simply blown away.

> *Compared to most of us in Europe, Chet Yorton and the other Americans were like special creations of science. Their bodies seemed totally ready – finished, polished. Mine was far from finished. I had just come to London with a big, muscular body.*

This was the beginning of a total rethink for Arnold, which as we well know would pay off – big time: the seventies were Arnold's decade in bodybuilding. He knew he had to have what Chet had.

What did he do that was different? The exercises he named were not in themselves different, but the way he did them was. His number of repetitions was higher. This helped separate the muscles and burn in the cuts.

Arnold clearly needed to change his routine from its early focus on strength and size. What Chet also had was a powerful, confident posing routine. We've already seen that Chuck Sipes failed to make the impact he should have done because of his disinterest in refining his posing routine; Arnold would not make that mistake.

Photographs of Yorton just don't do justice to the quality of his physique, according to fellow bodybuilder Bill Luttrell. Even some years later, after his competition days were well and truly over,

**everything* was [still] in perfect proportion, separated, and cut. I swear, no need to add or subtract an ounce anywhere. The finish to his physique had that very rare quality reminiscent of a thoroughbred horse or large cat. I don't want to overstate this too much, but unlike a lot of bodybuilders before or since, a build like that looks like it was made by the hand of God rather than Man – everything went together that well. Arnold, Dave, Pearl, Zane and very few others I can think of fall into that category.*

But it wasn't all just for show: Yorton was also very, very strong. He could squat and deadlift 600lb, and bench press around 500lb. Remember that it was only in the early 1950s that Doug Hepburn set the bench press record at 500lb (matched soon after by Reg Park), and not until 1967 that Pat Casey became the first man to press 600lb. Yorton's weird strength was fully on display in his weird training routine, which I'll lay out in as much detail as I can later. When it came to the bench press, for instance, in the off-season Yorton would press 225lb for 22 reps, then jump 100lb to 325lb and do another 22 reps. What's that I hear you say? 'Unbelievable'? No, not according to strength coach Bill Starr, who actually spotted for Yorton. 'I seriously doubt whether another bodybuilder—or strength athlete for that matter—in the world could duplicate such a feat.'

Everything about Chet Yorton's story seems designed to stretch credulity to breaking point – and beyond. And for the learned counsel of r/nattyorjuice, that would also include the crusade against steroids he took after his Mr Universe win, which led him on a Quixotic journey away from the mainstream for good. Chet's Damascus moment was similar to Chuck's. About two years before that famous night in London, Chet claims he was offered steroids by another 'top bodybuilder' at a gym, who waxed lyrical about the benefits; everybody was now taking them, he said. While Chet was initially intrigued, he was warned off by a doctor who told him of the potential side effects – gynecomastia, impotence, acne, hair loss, high blood pressure, etc. From then on, Chet began to speak out publicly. He came to see the rise of steroids as part of a broader destructive trend of immorality in bodybuilding, which compromised the integrity of bodybuilders as 'real' champions and role models; other shady practices included the sale of sexual favours for influence and an easy livelihood (sound familiar?) and political scheming in the governing bodies of the bodybuilding world (look up Arnold's comeback Olympia win, or Franco Colombo's second, in 1981, for example).

Chet had already incurred the wrath of the bodybuilding authorities by starring in the 1964 film *Muscle Beach Party* with Larry Scott and a number of other muscle men, including Dan 'Grizzly Adams' Haggerty. Although the film was a light-hearted affair about a group of bodybuilders taking over the secret surfing spot of the 'Beach Party Gang' (and one of seven *Beach Party* films), the Amateur Athletic Union did not see the funny side of it, and Chet was apparently singled out to be made an example of. The story goes – although Chet denies this – that he travelled to Chicago to compete in that year's Mr America contest, only to be turned away. He starred in another film, *Don't Make Waves*, with Dave Draper in 1966, the year when Chet won the NABBA Mr Universe and Draper the IFBB Mr Universe, but by this time Chet had stopped competing in AAU events, so the extra publicity could not harm his chances with that governing body at least.

After winning the 1966 Mr Universe, Chet chose to retire and focus on his supplement company, *Muscle Beach Supplements*, and his pool-cleaning business, which could boast Ronald Reagan and many of the Hollywood glitterati as customers. In 1972, he moved from California to Las Vegas and opened a gym called The Body Shop. After a few years, he was convinced he had what it took to compete again, and decided to enter the 1975 Mr Universe. Now his public stance on steroid use would apparently come back to bite him in his well-developed behind, as he lost – many say undeservingly – to self-admitted steroid user Boyer Coe. That loss was the final straw, and so the same year he founded the Natural Bodybuilder's Association, the first association to test for drug use at every competition. In his speech at its first annual competition, he pointed to the competitors and said, 'See, friends, these are the real champions.' He competed a few more times against untested competitors, including for rival breakaway governing bodies, but ultimately without success. In 1981, he launched the magazine *Natural Bodybuilding*. His contributions to natural bodybuilding were recognised in 2004 by the Organization of Competitive Bodybuilders, which awarded the first ever annual Yorton Cups to its male and female champions.

Even if Yorton's story isn't a true example of the outer limits of natural human potential for muscle growth, there remains much to be inspired by. The next time you complain about having an inauspicious start to your lifting career – *I wish I'd started lifting earlier / I wish my parents had fed me better / I wish I'd known then what I know now* – just picture young Chet, his legs broken and torn from their sockets, his arm sliced to pieces, a big piece of glass in his eye, sitting unconscious in that car for half an hour until the police arrived; if that isn't an inauspicious start – well, I don't know what is (maybe falling headfirst from a plane without a functioning parachute?). It certainly wasn't kvetching or finger-pointing that got him out of his wheelchair and onto the winner's podium at the Mr Universe eight years later…

… or that has kept him on the stage, even into his seventh decade. Although it's difficult to find out information about Chet these days (as far as I know he's still alive), there's a photo of him posing on stage at 67, and still looking more TST (thick, solid and tight) than most lifters half his age. 'The first seventy years were easy', he said on his seventieth birthday, 'but the next seventy are going to be a bitch'.

A triumph over adversity that would have killed or at the very least crippled a lesser man, Chester 'Chet' Yorton's story is a testament to the human potential for self-transformation. As the 1964 article in *Strength and Health*, put it: 'Just like the ancient Egyptian mythological bird, the phoenix, that was consumed by fire and then arose out of its own ashes to fly away and live another long life, so Chester Yorton climbed out of his own severely shattered bones to transform himself.'

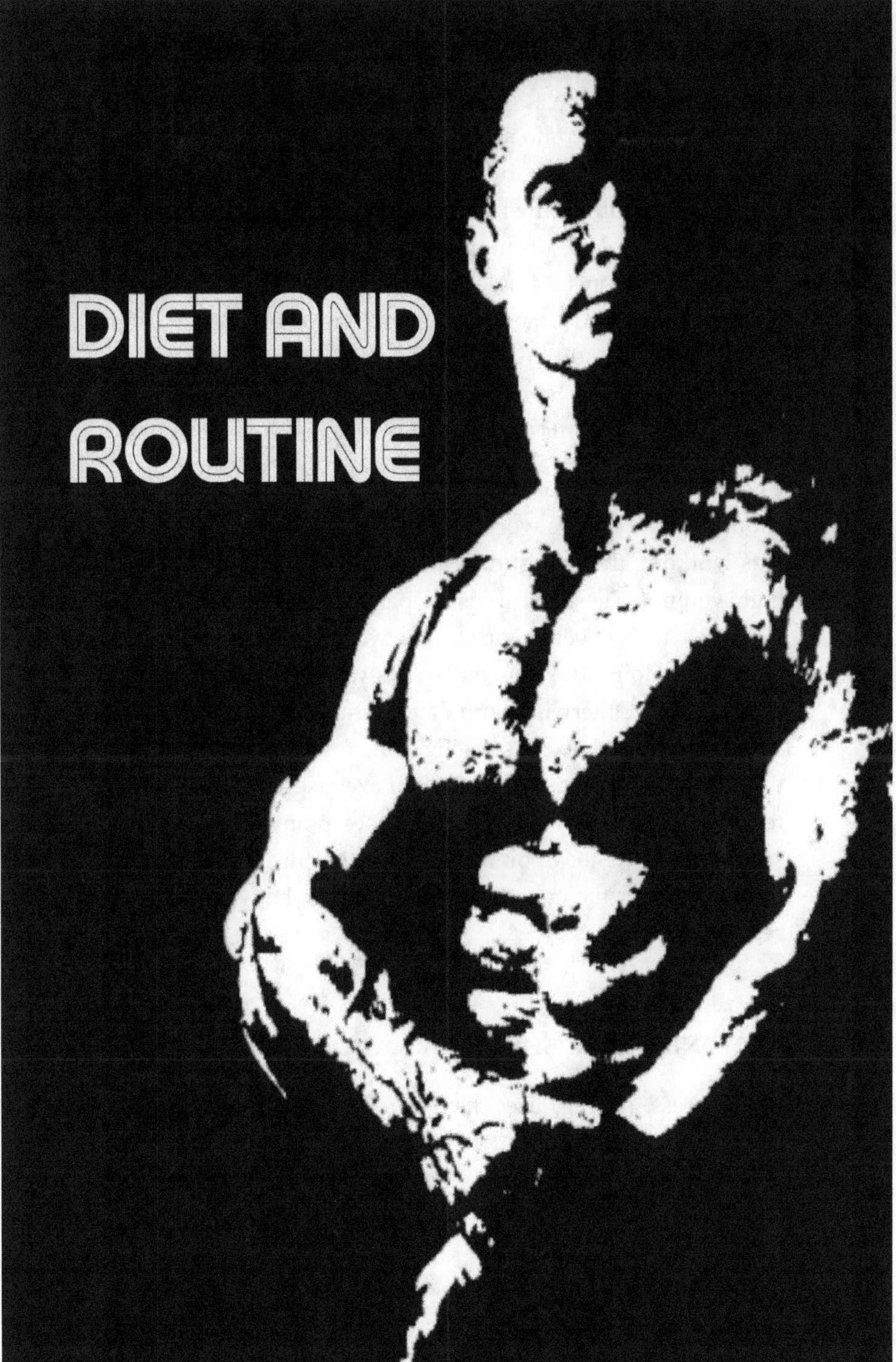

DIET AND
ROUTINE

If one thing's for certain about Chet Yorton, it's that he trained hard. If there's another thing, it's that his routine wasn't your average /fit/ routine either. Chet embraced a variety of training splits and rep ranges, from training six days a week to two-on-one-off, or even just a single session every five days in the off-season; I've already mentioned his 22-rep sets, which were combined with traditional rep ranges of 8-10, as well as greater numbers of reps for body parts like the calves, which were one of the many standouts that helped him defeat Arnold in 1966.

Chet's routine in preparation for a contest consisted of a chest, shoulders and triceps workout followed by a back biceps and legs workout, then a rest day, and repeat. The workouts were high volume. The most unusual part of this routine was his approach to the bench press. He would aim for 100 reps, usually by doing five sets of 22 reps with 315, followed by a one-rep max. Otherwise, both days featured exercises in the 8-10 rep range, each exercise being done for five sets, except for the calf and ab exercises. For the calf exercises, he would do 40 reps three times: the first with the toes pointed straight, the second with the toes pointed out and the third with the toes pointed in. For the crunches and leg raises, he would do 500 reps total each.

DAY ONE: CHEST, SHOULDERS AND TRICEPS

Bench press, lateral raises, bent-over lateral raises, overhead press, barbell front raise, tricep pushdowns, reverse grip dips, one-arm French press, tricep kickbacks, incline crunches and leg raises.

DAY TWO: BACK, BICEPS AND LEGS

Behind-the-neck pulldowns, wide-grip rows, reverse-grip rows, one-arm dumbbell rows, barbell curls, concentration curls, seated alternating dumbbell rows, standing dumbbell curls, squats, hack squats, leg curls, leg extensions, standing calf raises, incline crunches and leg raises.

Notice the use of classic exercises like the French press (or lying tricep extension) and behind-the-neck pulldowns.

It was during the off-season that Chet favoured his most unusual routine: a full body workout every five days consisting of two sets of 22 reps of squats, overhead press, bench press and deadlift.

The value of high-rep sets deserves some comment. High-rep exercises, especially high-rep squats, were an essential part of the routines of many Golden Age bodybuilders. High-rep squats, in particular, have long been touted with amazing anabolic effects; Randall Storrsen, for instance, author of the 1989 book *Super Squats*, claimed that a six-week routine of 20-rep squats could lead to up to 30lb of muscle growth, with growth not being limited to the legs but extending to the entire body. Twenty has been the magic number of reps since the 1930s, when Mark Berry, an American weightlifting coach, began to popularise high-rep squats in *Strength* magazine. One early high-rep squat routine was called the 'squats and milk' routine, involving 20-rep sets of squats and a GOMAD (gallon-of-milk-a-day) diet; note that the gallon of milk is not supposed to be the only food consumed, but is drunk in addition to a normal diet. Another early routine was devised by Joseph Hise, the so-called 'Daddy of the Squat', which he called 'breathing squats', because of the deep breathing required to complete one set; remember that Reg park performed these. The premise is simple, but at first sight confusing. The lifter must perform one set of 20 reps with a weight that is their 10-rep max. But that's impossible, surely? No: rest and deep breathing are used to allow the lifter to push on, through the pain, until they have completed 20 reps. Once the lifter hits ten reps, they must take a series of up to five deep breaths before the next repetition, and so on until they reach 20 reps. A set might, as a result, last as much as five minutes.

Later on, another daddy of the squat, the Quadfather himself, Tom Platz would insist on doing high-rep sets of squats. He claims that it was only when he started doing them that he began to build the freaky legs he is so famous for. On occasion, he was known to squat 225 for 100 reps, which took around ten minutes to complete. Here is his description of how it felt to finish a set of high-rep squats.

> *My heart rate soared upward and I found myself gasping for air. In a way, that sensation frightened me. I would fall to the floor, place the magical towel over my eyes, and ask myself, what if my heart does not slow down? I saw stars. My legs felt as if someone was stabbing knives into them.*

Not everybody is an advocate of high reps. According to our favourite tetchy uncle Mark Rippetoe, high reps usually become sloppy reps as fatigue sets in, hence his advocacy of five reps as a compromise between max strength and volume; with five reps, you won't feel the fatigue until *after* you put the bar down, or so the theory goes. Truth is, this argument can very simply be disproved by watching the famous video of Platz squatting 525lb for 23 reps, in his contest with the powerlifter Fred Hatfield; every single crushing rep is performed with a full range of motion and perfect – PERFECT – form.[3] If you're going to use higher reps with, say, the squat, build up to it gradually and don't compromise on form. Although Platz was beaten by Hatfield in terms of overall strength, he knocked him out of the park on the high-rep portion of the contest, because high reps were an essential part of his training, whereas maximum strength was the emphasis of Hatfield's. Don't think that you can squat weight X for 50 reps just because a rep calculator app tells you that you can.

The value of high-rep sets for overhead press, bench press and deadlift is less attested than for squats, but it's hard to argue with Yorton's results. With regard to the deadlift in particular, many argue, as Rippetoe does, that form is dangerously compromised and that the deadlift is too taxing on the central nervous system to be effective at higher rep ranges. You'll just have to find out for yourself.

As far as Chet's diet goes, that 1964 article in *Strength and Health* gives the most detailed description of Chet's diet and the general principles he followed. During heavy training, he would increase his food intake to match his exercise,

---

[3] Word is that Tom Platz managed 635 for 15 reps during his training for the 1986 Mr Olympia.

consuming six meals a day; when not in heavy training, he would stick to three meals a day.

> *He usually eats six to eight eggs for breakfast and two glasses of raw milk, plus soybean powder with brewer's yeast. For luncheon he has a light snack of one pound of rare ground beef, some vegetables and a gelatin salad plus his usual two glasses of raw milk, soybean powder and yeast. And for dinner he devours one pound of liver, chicken or steak, or sometimes fish, together with lots of vegetables and a salad, and as usual soybean powder, brewers [sic] yeast and two glasses of raw milk.[4]*

> *He obviously has remarkable metabolism. And I might also add that he eats no salt or other seasonings, no starches or dough; never tastes potatoes, bread, noodles, or cake, pie, ice cream, candy, gum or soda drinks.*

Eggs, raw milk, organ meat, lean muscle meat, fish and a bit of veg – barring the milk and veg, Chet could easily have been on a latter-day keto or paleo diet. Strict keto or not, it's clear that Chet was not consuming the generally recommended amount of carbohydrates for a bodybuilder looking to put on massive

---

[4] Brewer's yeast was very popular in the 1950s and 1960s health and fitness community, mainly for its vitamin and protein content. Vince Gironda was a famous advocate. The chromium in brewer's yeast may also have benefits for those with insulin sensitivity. By 'gelatin salad', a leaf salad with flavoured gelatin is probably meant. These were very common in American cooking of the time. Gelatin consumption has many benefits for the gut, skin and joints.

amounts of mass. 'Complex carbohydrates should make up the bulk of your daily calorie intake' (strengthandhealth.com) / 'The specific guidelines for a bodybuilding diet include from 55 to 60% of calories from carbohydrates, 25 to 30% from protein and 15 to 20% from fat' (nuts.com) / 'Most bodybuilders consume around 50% of total calories from carbs' (mensjournal.com). Although many classic bodybuilders and strength athletes have built tremendous physiques and physical strength on a simple meat and potatoes diet in vast quantities – and it's not a coincidence that many of them, like the Swedish brothers Magnus and Torbjörn Samuelsson, are or were also farmboys – Chet, by contrast, was shunning potatoes and other complex carbohydrates at a time when few others, except Vince Gironda, were doing so. Unlike with Gironda, the source of Chet's dietary ideas on carbohydrate restriction is unclear. Gironda's dietary ideas were not merely the result of his own experiments or anecdotes from others, but came from a reading in a wide variety of subjects, including scientific papers and also accounts of explorers like Vilhjalmur Stefansson who had spent time in the Arctic Circle with the Inuit, observing and following their high fat and protein diet. Gironda may also have read William Holston's 1963 article in the *California Historical Society Quarterly* on 'the Diet of the Mountain Men', whose entirely meat-based diet had shown that 'a predominantly raw, fresh meat bill of fare, supplemented with liberal quantities of fat, is one of the most healthful regimens that an individual can eat'. While Chet's physique alone should constitute a decisive intervention in the 'low carb can't build muscle' debate, I suspect the interminable discussion on r/ketoscience will remain just that.

It's clear, however, that Chet wasn't above cheating, especially when he was on the road, as an English friend of his recounts.

> *At 9pm that evening Chet was concerned that he hadn't had a workout for about 5 days with travelling and wanted to look well for his posing display the next day so I took him to my gym and he worked out for over 3 hours. By this time it had turned midnight and all the while he was worried that my wife might have gone to bed without leaving us some food. Not to worry she left all kinds of cold meats: ham, beef, chicken, eggs, tuna, salad, whole wheat bread – a whole tableful of food. I had a fairly normal plateful and Chet scarfed the rest and believe me I've never seen anyone eat as much food – he didn't leave a crumb!*

On this occasion, at least, he was happy to taste bread. But in the grand scheme of cheating, this is pretty austere, and bears no resemblance to the ~~Rack~~ Rock Dwayne Johnson's weekly Krispie Kreme and pancake binges.

Most of us would instinctively avoid anything soy, because of its phytoestrogenic properties, anti-nutrient content and the poor biological value of the protein it contains (a value of 74 by contrast with 100 for whole egg, #raweggnationalism). Soy was a common early protein powder of the 1950s and 1960s, and it shouldn't be forgotten that, long before Soylent, soy beans were thought of as a miracle food, mainly as a result of the nineteenth-century Austrian botanist Friedrich Haberland. The demands of the food shortages, especially protein shortages, during the interwar years after 1918 made soy cultivation especially attractive to European nations. Adolf Hitler, history's most famous vegetarian, was an aggressive proponent of soy. Hitler dreamed of replacing all German meat consumption with soy beans, which were dubbed 'Nazi beans', and during the Second World War, forced soybean cultivation on south-eastern Europe; soy-based rations were also given to Nazi soldiers. The soy didn't seem to harm their performance much either.

Another rich source of phytoestrogens Chet appears to have consumed on a regular basis was beer; although he moderated his consumption when he was training. While he lived in California, at a beach house in Malibu, he held regular parties several times a month. Both Arnold and Franco Columbo are known to have attended. Of the former, Jerry Brainum, of the Dave Draper forum, tells an amusing story.

I knew Chet Yorton, too. I have never seen any man drink as much alcohol as Chet did and walk normally. He favored 6-packs of Colt 45 malt liquor, and quarts of beer. I once attended a victory party Chet threw for himself at his Malibu home. At the party, I hung out with a then unknown fellow named Arnold Schwarzenegger who had recently arrived in this country. Arnold got drunk imbibing the copious beer that flowed at Yorton's bash. He tried to pick up a few women at the party – and was rejected every time. His come-on was quite crude in those days, made even worse by his intoxication. I still recall what he said to me after a few rejections: "I can't [believe] these women are rejecting me – they all look like a dog's dinner!

Chin up, Arnold: you can't always be numero uno.

In conclusion, it's most likely that Chet came to his ideas about training and dieting through trial and experiment more than through detailed research, unlike Gironda. No Golden Age bodybuilder, in their routine or diet, better embodies the Faustian spirit of the sport than Chet Yorton. At once experimenter and experiment, sculptor and sculpture, Chet was not afraid to find and then stick with what worked for him, regardless of what others around him were doing. Gymbros, take not